THE PLANT-BA

HOW IT'S GOING TO CHANGE

LIFE

TO Amanda
"The Knowledge of the truth
is power"

Olivier Mankondo

DEDICATIONS

To my wife, Mireille, who somehow managed to be nothing but supportive. This book is also dedicated to my children, Stevie, Olivia, David and Oliver – whose help made it possible – as well as my brother, Luc.

TABLE OF CONTENTS

ABOUT THE AUTHOR

Olivier Mankondo is a motivational speaker and a weight loss and wellness coach. He has been on a plant-based nutrition since 2016. He happened to be watching a program which showed how animal products aren't designed for the human mechanism. He applied this newfound knowledge in his life and was able to cure himself of high blood pressure, pre-diabetes, severe headaches, chest pains, painful joints, back pains, abscesses, and dandruff, without the use of any medication. Before adopting a plant-based nutrition and applying the newfound knowledge, Olivier Mankondo weighed 100 kilos (15½ stone) and lost 35 kilos (5½ stone) in 9 months, without surgery or physical exercises (gyms, bootcamps, etc.). After the change in his diet and lifestyle, Olivier's health has been optimal and he has never been sick for a single day.

INTRODUCTION

We have noticed that 70% of the world's population is sick. And when I say that 70% is sick, it doesn't necessarily mean that they're hospitalised; it just means that they're on some sort of prescribed medication by their doctors. If we add the number of people who auto-medicate, this number would be even higher. There's a study that suggests that 95% of us are sick. Even when we look at babies when they're born, after a week or two, they start being sick as well. This is really abnormal. If we look in the forest, we'll notice that the animal kingdom is doing far better than us, as there are no vets over there. The knowledge that I'm going to share in this book might appear a little bit unconventional for some, but I've done extensive research on the human mechanism and I'll speak as well from my personal experience. I used to weigh 100 kilos (15½ stone) and I've been able to lose 35 kilos (5½ stone) in 9 months. My health wasn't good, either, and I had loads of chronic diseases. I have also been able to cure myself of those diseases and my health is optimal now, so I know what I'm talking about. And those who will follow diligently the knowledge spread in this book will be able to reap the same benefits that I have. I would like the readers, as well, to use this book as a starting point to start their own research, too, to increase their knowledge, as knowledge is power.

PART I

For any machine to work in an optimal way, it needs the correct fuel. If you have a diesel car, you'll need to put diesel in it. If not, you're asking for trouble. For some reason, people seem to think that this law doesn't apply to the human mechanism. They think that we can eat anything and expect to be in good health and this is totally false. Now, we will look at the human mechanism and see what fuel it was really designed for. And to be able to do this, I'll have to compare the carnivores and the herbivores and see to whom human beings relate to.

1. COMPARISON BETWEEN THE CARNOVIRES AND THE HERBIVORES

If we look in the mouth region, we can see that the carnivores have two piercing canines, they've got shorter incisors and their molars are not developed. The carnivores have only got one movement in their jaws: they don't chew their food – they can only cut and swallow. But we if we look at the herbivores, their canines are not developed, their incisors and their molars are developed, and they've got two movements in their mouths. They have to cut and chew their food. If we look at human beings, they have to chew their food just like herbivores. In this instance, you can see that human beings relate more to herbivores rather than carnivores.

If we look at the bite force, for the dogs, it's between 300-400 PSI; for the lions and the tigers, it's 800-900 PSI; for hyenas it's above 1000 PSI. And for humans, it's only 135-150 PSI.

When we look at carnivores, they lick up water when they want to drink, while human beings suck up their water just like herbivores. Here, again, human beings relate more to herbivores.

Carnivores pant while herbivores sweat through their skin. Human beings, too, sweat through their skin, just like herbivores.

The length of gestation for all carnivores is inferior or equal to 15 weeks: the gestation period for the wolf is 9 weeks; for the cheetah, it's 13 weeks; for the lion, it's 15 weeks. But if we look at the gestation period for herbivores/frugivores, it's superior or equal to 34 weeks: the gestation period for the bison is 40 weeks; the horse is 47 weeks; the chimpanzee is 34 weeks; the gorilla is 36 weeks; the orangutan is 38 weeks; and for humans, it's 40 weeks. Again, in this instance, human beings relate more to herbivores, not carnivores.

The carnivores have got a shorter gestation period and they've got multiple-birth. For example, a dog will have 5-6 puppies at the same time. And when these carnivores are born, for the first 2 weeks, they're blind. The herbivores/frugivores have got a longer gestation period and they've got single-birth. For example, a cow will have only 1 calf; an elephant will only have only 1 baby. And when all of the above herbivores are born, they can see straight away. For us humans, we have single-birth, as well, and rarely twins (or triplets). When our babies are born, they can see, straight away. In this instance, again, we are just like herbivores.

If we look at the digestive tract, herbivores have got long intestines, which are roughly 6 times the length of their bodies. On the contrary, the carnivores have got shorter intestines, which are roughly 3 times the length of their bodies. For us humans, we've got longer intestines, just like herbivores. Our intestines are 9 metres or 27 feet long. Once again, we fall in the same category as herbivores.

Carnivores have got very powerful kidneys, as the meat gets transformed into uric acid, which they need powerful kidneys to get rid of.

The digestion process starts in the mouth region for the human beings and the herbivores. They've both got an enzyme called Ptyalin which enables the start of the digestion process. But you don't find this enzyme in any carnivores. Yet another similitude between the herbivores and the human beings.

From this comparison, you can clearly see that human beings are herbivores or mostly frugivores, and have got nothing in common with carnivores. To push this logic a little bit further, we share 99% of the same DNA with gorillas, but gorillas eat only fruits, vegetables and tender roots – they DO NOT eat meat. How come we share 99% of the same DNA but our diets are supposedly completely different?

2. THE BOWEL TRANSIT TIME

To understand what the wrong foods do to our system, we'll have to have a look at the bowel transit time. The bowel transit time is the time that a certain kind of food takes to pass through our system. So, if we eat fruit, it takes 3-4 hours to pass through our system; if we eat raw vegetables, it takes around 12 hours; if we eat cooked vegetables, it takes between 24 and 30 hours. But if we eat animal products like meat, fish and chicken, it takes 72 hours or 3 days to pass through our system. Meat passes through the system very slowly – that's why carnivores have got smaller intestines. Fruits and vegetables pass through the system very quickly – that's why human beings and herbivores have got longer intestines.

3. ANIMAL PRODUCTS

If we were designed to eat meat, then nature would've provided us with the tools. If a carnivore wants to kill its prey, it only needs its teeth and its claws. Why do us humans need knives, guns, etc. to kill, plus the fact that we'll need to cook it once we're done? With just our teeth and our hands, it's almost impossible to kill an animal. And even if we could, they would easily outrun us. Let's assume that you're lost in a forest. The first idea that comes to your mind, regarding food, is fruit – this is suggestive of our true nature. Nobody will try to catch a gazelle.

If we eat the wrong food for the first 20-25 years of lives, our body will manage (to a certain extent), but after that, it'll be overwhelmed. Like I said before, the animal products take around 3 days to pass through our system. If we were to put meat, fish and chicken outside during the summer for 3 days, these animal products would be in a state of decay. You'll see maggots, worms, flies, etc... If we look at the internal temperature of the average human being, you'll find that it'll be 36 degrees centigrade. So it's hot like a summer day. The rotting process that I described earlier is exactly what occurs inside your guts after ingesting some animal products. There's a rotting process taking place, and that's why people smell bad and have foul breath. People feel the need to mask that bad smell with perfume and deodorant, and people feel the need to brush their teeth as much as they want to get rid of that foul breath. A lot of people have been autopsied and they were able to find worms, maggots and impacted faeces in their colons – that's what happens when you have rotting matter lying around in your gut. When this rotting process is happening, there's an incredible amount of bacterial activity going on. The body will have to produce a lot of energy to try and reduce this number of bacteria, which is why people seem to constantly feel tired, always needing stimulants like coffee and energy drinks, despite them having a full-night's sleep. Animal products have got no fibre and create constipation. There are a lot of people who can spend 3-4 days, even a week without going to the toilet once. This is very detrimental to the human system. When you're constipated, the faecal matter will be reabsorbed into your bloodstream, and that's how we get all the chronic diseases such as:

. high blood pressure

. diabetes

. cancer

. Parkinson's

. Alzheimer's

. strokes

. arthritis

. and all the autoimmune diseases where the body destroys itself. These would include

. the inflammatory bowel disease

. multiple sclerosis

. lupus

. psoriasis

.celiac disease

.Type 1 diabetes

. rheumatoid arthritis.

According to the World Health Organisation, processed meat like salami, sausages, bacon and hotdogs cause cancer. Beef, lamb and pork have also been noted to possibly be carcinogens. Here are the dangers of processed meat:

. Colorectal cancer

. Heart disease

. Increased risk of death

. Prostate cancer

. Breast cancer

When you're constipated, it's like having a blocked toilet but still continuing to use it. Now imagine that your entire house is full of faecal matter. How will you be able to sustain life in these conditions? The premise is the same when describing how your cells are swimming in foul blood. It's impossible to have optimal health. We've also been told that chicken is very good. They call it "white meat." But did you know that poultry gives breast cancer, prostate cancer, colon cancer, brain cancer, obesity, heart attacks, diabetes, and more?

Meat promotes free radicals as well. Free radicals are unstable atoms which can damage cells, causing illness and aging.

In the forest, animals don't get sick unless they're attacked such as when males fight for females. There are no vets in the forest, but domesticated animals fall sick just like us, since they're not being fed the food that they were biologically designed for. Cats and dogs need to eat raw meat, but instead, we give them cooked food, biscuits, cookies, etc…You'll see these same animals suffering from blindness, cancer, multiple sclerosis, etc… In zoos, you'll see gorillas suffering from diabetes and high blood pressure (which is impossible to see them having when they're living in nature.) The cow eats grass, but they're given corn and meat powder, which is why you've heard of cows, in the past, suffering from the mad cow disease.

Apart from meat being a poison to the human system, all these animals are raised in appalling conditions like confined spaces with no sunlight, which becomes really difficult to sustain life in. They get loads of infections, which is why 70% of the antibiotics produced worldwide are used to treat these animals. And when we eat them, these antibiotics are passed to us. Antibiotics are very bad for the human mechanism, as they impair and destroy the bacterial flora in the intestines. 80% of the human immune system is located in the intestines. The role of the appendix is to repopulate your gut with good bacteria. Doctors have always thought that the appendix has no function in the body, however this is far from true: it helps strengthen and support your immune system. People with removed appendixes are 4 times more likely to have a reoccurrence of bacterial infection which causes diarrhea, fever, nausea and abdominal pains. They've got a 60% risk of developing colon cancer, as well.

The lifespan of a chicken is between 6 and 8 years, but when they're raised in these animal farms, they need to reach a weight of 2 kilos in 42 days; this never happens in nature. And because they're putting on weight this quickly, their fragile skeleton becomes incapable of supporting their weight. You'll find that lots of these chickens end up dying on the soil because other chickens peck them to death due to their dangerously large weight, they lose their ability to walk, quickly becoming an easy target for other chickens. Cannibalism outbreaks can be initiated by the injury of one chicken.

These animals know that they will be killed and thus begin to produce harmful chemicals which will be detrimental to our health.

70 billion land animals are killed every year, alone.

We have also been told that fish is very good for our health, but you should know that fish are loaded with mercury, which is a heavy metal that you should avoid at all costs. That's why they don't manufacture thermometers with mercury anymore. Mercury is so toxic that if you were to have spill, the fire brigade would have to be called and access to the building would be prohibited for 2-3 days. Mercury has a very toxic effect on the nervous system, the digestive system, the immune system, the lungs, the kidneys, the skin and the eyes. From this, you can really appreciate the deadliness of animal products.

4. DAIRY PRODUCTS

The dairy products are another deadly component which destroys our health. Human beings are the only organisms that drink the milk of another species. It doesn't happen anywhere else. You'll never see a cat drinking dogs milk or a goat drinking cow's milk. Every type of milk is specific to their respective species. For example, rabbit milk has 10 times more protein than human milk, since when the baby rabbit is born, its size needs to be doubled within the 1st week of its life, in order to sustain life. Seal milk is composed of 40% fat, as the baby seal needs to build up fat very quickly, considering how cold the north pole can get. Human milk has got lactalbumin, as we need to produce amino acids. Cow's milk has got casein, which is its primary element and isn't anywhere to be seen in human milk. Now you can see how each kind of milk is specific to its species.

A calf, when born, weighs 30 kilos (5 stone) and needs to triple its weight in 3 months – this is why cow's milk contains a lot of growth hormones and calcium because the calf will grow to be a large cow/bull. So when we drink milk, we receive too much calcium, which we rid ourselves of when we urinate, however this comes at the expense of some of the calcium that we actually needed. Cow's milk has too much phosphorus for humans, too, and to neutralise that phosphorus, our body will have to leech out calcium from our muscles, our bones and our teeth, which is how osteoporosis comes about (when your bones become brittle and you get inflamed joints). You can see how in countries where the milk intake is high, you'll have more instances of osteoporosis – this warrants people to walking aids, scooters, canes, etc...

These cows, as well, are milked all day long, which creates an infection called mastitis, which creates pus (this gets mixed up with the milk, even though they tell you that the milk will be pasteurized, but it makes no difference).

Human beings are the only species on Earth that drink milk even when they're adults. We produce an enzyme which enables us to digest the milk. When we reach 2-4 years old, this enzyme ceases to be produced, which suggests that we should stop drinking milk. And that's why 70% of the population is lactose intolerant – and when I say lactose intolerant, I don't necessarily mean that they'll suffer from strong allergic reactions. This can be manifested in a subtle way, like

. chronic fatigue,

. chronic inflammation,

. digestive problems, etc...

Here is a list of diseases caused by dairy products:

. Anemia

. Ear infections

. Appendicitis

. Eczema

. Asthma

. Osteoporosis

. Leukemia

. Multiple sclerosis

. Cancer

. Allergies

. Obesity

. Arthritis

. Lymphoma

. etc...

Because of all these growth hormones, boys and girls go through puberty very early, and they'll produce too much estrogen. Too much estrogen is linked to cancer and that's why you'll see girls having breast cancer, ovarian cancer, uterus cancer later on in life, and boy's having prostate cancer.

Eggs, too, are very bad for the human mechanism, as it's very high in cholesterol. This cholesterol will clog up your arteries and you'll have strokes, heart problems, etc...

There's a compound called lecithin in egg yolks which gets converted into chemical TMAO when in contact with your gut bacteria. A high level of TMAO is linked to heart attacks and strokes.

When we eat concentrated animal protein, the body will start producing a high level of hormone called insulin like growth factor 1 (IGF1). A high level of IGF1 is associated with an increase of cancer risk.

Good alternatives for cow's milk are soy milk (ensure that it's organic), almond milk, coconut milk and rice milk (consume in moderation).

5. PROCESSED FOOD

Another bad food for the human mechanism is the processed food which is essentially man-made food. These foods have been transformed and resemble nothing in nature. You find them in cartons, cans, bottles, etc... 51% of what people eat is processed food, 42% are animal products, and only 7% are fruit and vegetables. And in that 7%, most of the foods are potatoes to make French fries. These processed foods are full of flavourings, preservatives, additives and colourings, which are chemical substances not recognised by the human body and thus create havoc.

The processed foods will raise your risk of getting cancer, they are loaded with added sugar, sodium and fat, are designed to make you overeat and become addicted to them, and, of course, they're high in carbs and low in nutrients and fibres.

In this category, as well, you have white sugar, white rice and white flour, which are refined. To give them their white appearance, they're polished, which deprive them of their nutrients and vitamins, making them very toxic to the body. You need to eat brown rice, brown sugar and wholemeal brown flour instead.

You've also got aspartame, which is an artificial sweetener which is highly toxic and is a nerve poison. You'll find aspartame in 10,000 products in supermarkets. You find aspartame in commercial juices, soft drinks, chewing gum, sweets, canned food, cookies, biscuits, etc...Here are some side effects of aspartame:

. Muscle spasms

. Heart palpitations

. Weight gain

. Breathing difficulty

. Blindness

. Severe depression

. Seizures

. Obesity

. Testicular, mammary and brain tumours

. Sex dysfunctions

. Cancer

. Hyperactivity in children

. Birth defects including mental retardation

. Death

Here is a list of the foods with the most acidifying effects:

. Milk

. Meat products

. Tinned or frozen foods

. White bread

. Pasta and pastries made from bleached and refined flour

. Refined white sugar

. Alcoholic drinks

. Diet drinks

. Soft drinks

. Sport drinks

. Packaged fruit juices

. Processed breakfast cereals

. Ready-made cakes

. Crisps

. Hydrogenated oils

. Oils and fats

. Most fast/junk foods

The body needs lots of minerals (potassium, magnesium, iron, iodine, calcium, etc.) and you can only find them in the plant kingdom. Cancer cells need fat and sugar to thrive and cannot live in an oxygen-rich environment. When you eat animal products, your blood pH goes beneath 7 and your blood has difficulty circulating the oxygen, which then makes for a good field for cancer cells to develop (normal pH is between 7.35 and 7.4). If your diet is too acidic, the blood will be forced to use minerals that you get from your food. If no minerals are found in your food, the body will leech out minerals from your bones, teeth and muscles, and you'll suffer from inflammation of the joints.

PART II

6. THE TRANSFORMATION

Our body is electrical and works on micro electricity. You can only have this vital energy from live foods, which are fruit, vegetables, legumes, grains, nuts and seeds, contrary to the animal products and the processed foods. As soon as the animal is dead, the rotting process begins immediately, making them dead foods. You can't put canned food in soil and expect it to grow, because it's dead food. How can you feed a living body with dead food and expect it work in an optimal manner? If you've got a green banana, after a couple of days it'll become yellow (ripe), then after a week or so (provided that it doesn't get eaten) the rotting process starts. You can see, now, how bananas are living. There are even some vegetables that you can put in the fridge and they continue to grow, meaning that they're still living. You can take a seed from a fruit, put it in soil and you'll see it grow because it's alive. To conclude, dead food have got no life energy, therefore meaning that they can only produce death.

For people who are Christians, if you look in the bible, in Genesis 1:29 says "God also told them, look! I have given you every seed-bearing plant that grows throughout the earth, along with every tree that grows seed-bearing fruit. They will produce your food."

I have applied this statement to my life and I've experienced a tremendous transformation. I was just like everybody else – eating all the animal products, processed foods, fast foods, junk foods and dairy products I could find, and it seemed very normal to me. But at that time, I was suffering from loads of diseases. I had high blood pressure, back pains, painful joints, severe headaches, abscesses, dandruff, chest pains and I was pre-diabetic. I was told by doctors that I'd be on medication for the rest of my life. My weight was 100 kilos (15½ stone) at the time but when I decided to go on a plant-based nutrition, I saw tremendous changes. Within 9 months, I lost 35 kilos (5½ stone) and since that time, my weight hasn't increased. My BMI was 32 – it's 22 now. All my ailments are completely gone. I haven't got high blood pressure, anymore. At its highest, my blood pressure was 167/110 (normal blood pressure is 140/80), and now, it's 124/70. I'm no longer pre-diabetic. At that time, my blood sugar was at 41. If you reach 42, you are declared fully diabetic. Today, 3 years after I went on a plant-based nutrition, my blood sugar is at 37. I have no more headaches, no more back and chest pains, no dandruffs, no abscesses; I'm completely cured.

My wife was overweight, too. Her weight was 109 kilos (17 stone) and after embracing the plant-based nutrition, her weight plummeted to 70 kilos (11½ stone). And the beauty of losing weight naturally, is that you're not left with loose skin, as opposed to when you go under the knife or when you exercise intensively.

One of my sons had eczema for 11 years. He was prescribed all sorts of medications, but to no avail. But when he went on this plant-based nutrition, it only took 2 weeks for the eczema to disappear completely.

My brother, as well, was more or less like me. He had high blood pressure, headaches, psoriasis and he was pre-diabetic, too. The doctor told him that he would have the psoriasis for the rest of his life. He already had that for 8 years and was put on very strong steroids, but there were no changes. His weight was 103 kilos (16½ stone) but when I introduced him to this plant-based nutrition, the same transformation that occurred to me, occurred to him, as well. His weight went down to 68 kilos (11 stone). He was cured of all his ailments, including the psoriasis promised he would have for the rest of his life.

You can now see the power of nutrition. For all of us, our conditions have been reversed with no medications, whatsoever.

And since I've been on this plant-based nutrition, I've not been sick for a single day for the past 3 years – not even a cough, a cold, the flu, etc...

7. WHAT IS DISEASE?

When we're sick, it's a way for our body to tell us that we've violated the laws that govern it, and it's trying to ask us to fix the mistake that we made.

There is only one disease. People will call it cancer, high blood pressure, diabetes, multiple sclerosis, Parkinson's, Alzheimer's, etc... but essentially, the disease is the malfunctioning of our cells. There are only 2 causes of disease: toxicity and deficiency.

We put toxins in our bodies by eating animal products, dairy products, processed foods, the cosmetic products that we apply to our faces and skins. We also put toxins in our bodies by the way we think and act.

We are deficient because we don't give the body the food it was designed for and it doesn't get the nutrients and vitamins it needs. That's why the body will keep giving you signals that it needs those nutrients, and it's also why people are always hungry.

And by continuing to give the body the wrong foods, people become obese or overweight.

In conventional medicine, when someone is ill, they will give them some pills, which will only suppress the symptoms without actually addressing the root cause. For example, when you get a cough or catch a cold, people don't ask themselves why their body is giving themselves such a problem. And because those symptoms are unpleasant, people will take medication to stop that. And the job that your body was trying to do to get rid of all these toxins will be stopped and they'll be buried in your tissues. And the more you repeat this process, these acute diseases will be transformed into chronic diseases.

Another example of this behaviour is that when you have high blood pressure, the doctor will put you on medication straight away without trying to find out the root cause of the problems - they will only treat the symptoms.

But let me explain to you why most of us suffer from high blood pressure: when you start eating food that isn't designed for this body, the food will start creating lesions in the arteries. Your body, in its wisdom, will want to heal these lesions, and will start producing cholesterol to patch those lesions. And the more you eat the wrong food, the more the body will produce cholesterol. But the doctors, in their ignorance, will put you on medication to reduce the cholesterol which is helping you to reduce the damage you're doing to your arteries. Because of this cholesterol build-up, you'll see that the diameter of your arteries will start narrowing and the blood will have a hard time flowing easily. And because your body is super intelligent, it'll create a coping mechanism to deal with the abuse you're inflicting on it. It will then raise your blood pressure so that the blood will still be able to go everywhere, in spite of the blockage caused by the cholesterol. Again, due to their ignorance, doctors will do their best to decrease the blood pressure, while your body is doing something vital for your survival.

Wouldn't it be better to deal with the root cause to try and solve the situation? That's exactly what I did. I stopped eating those damaging foods not designed for the human mechanism and replaced them with nutrient-dense foods. My body didn't find the need to produce cholesterol anymore, which lead to the opening up of all my arteries. My blood was now able to flow without any obstructions. And voila! I was cured of my high blood pressure. Isn't that easier than being put on medication for the rest of your life?!

And the men's erectile dysfunction problem has got the same root cause, which is eating food not designed for this body. As I've said before, the narrowing of the arteries will obstruct the blood flow. And to have an erection, you need sufficient blood in your penis. By removing all the damaging foods, your blood pressure will be normal and you'll be able to sustain and erection. But in conventional medicine, if you have an erectile dysfunction problem, they will put you on some medication, and usually it's Viagra. But here are some Viagra side effects:

. Priapism (it's a condition where the erection will not go away after 4 hours - if that happens, your penis will be damaged permanently)

. Loss of vision in one or both eyes

. Sudden hearing loss or decrease

. Upset stomach

. Rashes

. Heart attacks

. Strokes

. Potentially death

This is exactly the same with Type 2 diabetes. But let's see why people suffer from diabetes. In conventional medicine, they will tell you that the sugar and carbohydrates are responsible for diabetes. That's why they will prohibit people from even eating fruits.

But here is the difference between the refine sugar and the fruit sugar. The refined sugar is bio-available, which means that it goes straight into your bloodstream and will create spikes of insulin. By creating spikes of insulin like that, your system will collapse in the long run. On the other hand, fruit sugar is not bio-available. Before entering your bloodstream, the fruit will first go into your stomach and after being digested, the nutrients will be absorbed in the small intestines. And only then will the sugar be available in your bloodstream, and your body will only have to produce a very small amount of insulin. This is the major difference between refined sugar and fruit sugar.

Let's see, now, what actually creates Type 2 diabetes. When you eat animal products, you will start having fat around your cells. Normally when you have sugar in your bloodstream, insulin acts like a key. In the presence of sugar in your bloodstream, your body will produce insulin, which will open up the cells and the sugar will be able to make its way into the cells. But when you get fat around your cells, the insulin won't be able to signal the cells to open up and the more you eat sugar, the more insulin will be produced. And because of the fat around the cells, the sugar will go nowhere but stay in your bloodstream. That's how you become insulin resistant and you're inevitably declared diabetic.

To reverse this condition, stop eating animal products. The fat around the cells will go away, the insulin will be able to send the signal for the cells to open up, you won't have a build-up of sugar in your bloodstream anymore, and you'll be cured of your diabetes. Simple, isn't it? You don't need medication to treat your diabetes.

I was eating animal products and my blood sugar was at 41. I have stopped eating animal products and eating tons of fruits and my blood sugar is now at 37. Understand that the fruit sugar has got nothing to do with the diabetes. It's the animal products.

Speaking of which, why do people suffer from acid reflux? When you have acid reflux, doctors will give you anti-acid because they think that you have too much acid. But the truth of the matter says otherwise. When people eat the wrong food, it starts damaging the mucus of the stomach lining. As an intelligent reaction from the body, it's going to reduce the acid in the stomach to avoid damaging it further. And because the food doesn't get digested properly anymore, you get acid reflux, since, from time to time, the lower esophageal sphincter (LES) relaxes inappropriately. If you want to fix the issue, stop eating the food that's damaging your stomach lining. Your body will repair itself and the production of acid will regulate, resolving your problem. You need to address the root cause and not the symptoms.

When supressing the symptoms by using medication, you'll feel better for a short period of time, but the disease will come back, as you will have not addressed the root cause.

I will use an analogy to try and explain this: let's say that you're driving your car and suddenly a light starts flashing in your dashboard, letting you know that you've got an oil leakage. You take your car to the mechanic but he just takes out a fuse. The flashing light stops and he tells you that your car has been fixed. When you take medication, the symptom disappears just like the flashing lights after they take out the fuse, but it doesn't mean that the car is fixed. If you continue to drive the car, the oil will continue to leak and one day, your car engine will stop working and your car will be good for the scrapyard. If you take medication, the symptoms will disappear, but the disease will continue to advance in silence. And one day, all of a sudden, you'll have a heart attack, a stroke, cancer or maybe you just drop dead. And people will ask "How can they die so suddenly?" If you opt for surgery and get an organ removed, the disease will come back in another form or in another organ, as the cause which made your organ to malfunction has not been dealt with. If you want to have an organ transplanted, your immune system will reject the new organ. That's why you'll have to undergo immunosuppressive therapy, which will weaken your immune system and you'll be open to all sorts of diseases. Medication essentially just increases the toxicity that made you sick in the first place. All medication without exception has got side effects and will make you sicker and sicker, killing you in the long run.

Here are some side effects of a flu medication that you can buy over the counter:

"Allergic reactions which may be severe, such as itching (sometimes with swelling of the mouth or face)"

. "Skin rash or peeling"

. "Breathing problems"

. "Unexplained bruising or bleeding"

. "Reoccurring fevers or infections"

. "Nausea, sudden weight loss, loss of appetite and yellowing of the eyes and skin"

. "Visual disturbances"

. "Unusually fast pulse rate or irregularly heartbeat"

. "Difficulty passing water"

. "Raised blood pressure"

. "Headache"

. "Dizziness"

. "Difficulty sleeping"

. "Nervousness"

. "Anxiety"

. "Diarrhea"

You can see for yourself all of the huge side effects of a seemingly harmless medication that you could get over the counter.

The leading cause of death in the world is heart disease. In 2nd place is cancer, and, in some countries, medication and medical intervention is the 3rd leading cause of death.

If you're suffering from high blood pressure, the medication will lower your blood pressure, but it's a poison for your liver, your heart and your kidneys. Here are some side effects of the blood pressure medication:

. Sexual impotence

. Cough

. Diarrhea

. Constipation

. Feeling tired

. Feeling nervous

. Headaches

. Nausea

. Sleepiness

. Lethargy

. etc.

But I want to be clear, here. I'm not asking anyone to completely shut themselves off from their medication. I'm trying to say that if you go on a plant-based nutrition where you only eat wholefood, you're not going to really need medication anyways, as you'll have an alkaline body where pathogens cannot develop. I'm not implying, either, that medicine is useless. Conventional medical treatment like reconstruction surgery is very good for dealing with trauma, or if you're involved in an accident, you can use conventional medicine to deal with your burns, cuts, broken limbs, gunshot wounds, etc... Yes, medicine is very good for that, but certainly not for treating chronic diseases.

For example, for the cancer treatment, conventional medicine uses chemotherapy, radiotherapy and surgery. But you've never been told that chemotherapy destroys your immune system, which is your body's only line of defence. It's like having ants in your house and you want to get rid of them, but instead of dealing with them normally, you decide to drop a bomb on your house. You'll destroy everything. It's the same with chemotherapy: it destroys both the cancerous cells AND the good cells, leaving your body vulnerable to any and all attacks. Here are some chemotherapy side effects:

. Brain damage

. Constipation

. An increase risk of picking up infections

. Itchy skin

. Hearing loss

. Loss of sensation in your hands, fingers and toes

. Kidney and bladder damage (some people will stay in diapers for the rest of their lives)

. Heart and lung damage

. Hair loss

. Fatigue

. Nausea and vomiting

. Diarrhoea

. Mouth ulcers

. etc.

Chemotherapy gives you MORE cancer, as the chemical substances used are carcinogens.

Chemotherapy is used to kill cancer cells so that tumours don't grow anymore. But a new study found out that chemo could help the cancer spread and lead to more aggressive types.

In the short term, it was found that the tumours were shrinking with that treatment but the chemo were increasing the chances of the cancer cells to migrate to another part of the body and trigger a repair which will allow those cancer cells to grow back stronger. This is according to a team of US researchers.

A study was made and 90% of the oncologists said that if they had cancer, they'd never have chemotherapy, since they know of the devastating effects of such treatments. And you've not been told, as well, that only 5% of people survive cancer and 95% die – not necessarily from the cancer itself, but mostly from the side effects of its supposed "treatment."

You'll certainly ask yourself "Why have we never been told this? Why don't they talk about this on TV, in the newspaper or on the radios?" What you need to know is that the pharmaceutical industry is the biggest business in the world. It's not diamonds, gold, oil or anything else you've been made to believe. The pharmaceutical industries make money off of sick people and, like I said at the beginning of this book, 70% of the world's population is sick. There's no need for them to tell you to go on a plant-based nutrition to be in good health. Who's going to buy all these billions of pills if they told you the truth? In fact, if they did that, the economy would collapse. You can even see all the attached businesses to Big Pharma.

We are in 2019 and, for the past four years, I've not taken a single pill. Imagine everyone not needing medication. Like I've just mentioned, this would mean the collapse of the entire system.

They need to keep you under the illusion that medication is needed to be in good health, while nobody gets better, especially if you have chronic diseases. They will add more and more medication and your situation will not get better but, in fact, it'll get worse until your body won't be able to take it anymore.

PART III

8. WHAT TO DO TO BE IN GOOD HEALTH

If you want to be in good health, there's a few things that you'll have to do on a daily basis.

A.) You will have to stop eating animal products, dairy products and processed foods, as they're not designed for human consumption.

B.) You will have to start filtering your tap water, as it contains fluoride and chlorine. They are both linked to cancer.

If you have a look at toothpaste packet, you'll find that it says you need to use a small amount. According to the packet itself, if you ingest the toothpaste, you'll need to seek medical attention. Why would you seek medical attention for something that is supposedly good for you? You need to ask yourself the question.

Sodium fluoride

. kills rodents

. causes cancer

. lowers your IQ

. causes apathy

. and was used by Nazis in the concentration camps.

. It creates bone weakness

. inhibits melatonin production

. impairs your immune system

. lowers your sex drive and causes infertility.

C.) You need to stop using cream, hairspray and cosmetic products which include toxic chemicals. Sodium laureth/lauryl sulfate (SLS) is present in these cosmetic products and creates skin irritation, organ toxicity and cancer. It's an additive that allows cleaning products to foam. Nearly 16,000 studies mentioned the toxicity of SLS, a surfactant, detergent and emulsifier used in thousands of cosmetic products and industrial cleaners. SLS has also been linked to nitrosamines, potent carcinogens that cause your body to absorb nitrates (which are known to be carcinogenic, as well).

What you should know, as well, is that what you put on your skin can be more dangerous than what you eat. When you put chemicals on your skin or hair – such as getting your hair dyed – may actually be worse than eating them. When you eat something, the enzymes in your saliva and stomach help to break it down and flush it out of your system. However, when you put these chemicals onto your skin, they're absorbed straight into your bloodstream without being filtered at all, which means that they'll go directly to your organs. You have paraben in those cosmetic products, which is, too, linked to cancer. They use paraben to prevent bacteria from accumulating in those products in order to increase their shelf lives.

You have another product called BPA (Bisphenol A), which causes cancer since it messes up your estrogen. You find BPA in products like:

. plastic containers

. canned food,

. toiletries

. hygiene products for women

. contact lenses

. thermal printer receipts

. Household electronics

. and dental filling sealants.

The perfume and deodorant are loaded with aluminium, which is linked to Alzheimer's. The department of neurology and psychiatry at St. Louis University said that aluminium may cause liver toxicity and lead to degenerative symptoms, including Alzheimer's. Therefore, you need to avoid these sources of aluminium toxicity, which would be

. the commercial deodorant

. commercial baking powder

. aluminium foil

. aluminium cookware

. vaccines and chemtrails.

Vaccines contain known carcinogen formaldehyde, which is used to embalm dead people. Almost every single vaccine on the market has some amount of aluminium in it, and some more than others. Apart from formaldehyde and aluminium, you have mercury, as well, in those vaccines, which create a deadly mixture. The mercury-based thimerosal as a preservative in vaccines, has been associated with autism. Despite the evidence, mercury is still added to vaccines at a completely unsafe level, considering the fact that it is a neurotoxin. This is why you've most likely noticed that the number of autistic kids has skyrocketed.

A vaccine that contains mercury may not show any damage for several months. Increasing evidence shows that chronic diseases such as rheumatoid arthritis, encephalitis, multiple sclerosis, leukemia and other forms of cancer are all linked to vaccinations administered in the early stages of life.

D.) Stop eating refined salt. The table salt used by most people is heavily processed and horrible for our health and will dehydrate your body. Other side effects include weight gain and high blood pressure.

You can use instead the sea salt, celtic salt or the Himalayan salt.

E.) You've got to stop eating microwaved food. When we put food inside of a microwave, the molecules that compose the food will begin to move at an incredible speed and the friction between those molecules is what creates the heat. When you take the food out of the microwave, it'll still look like food, but its molecular structure will be completely destroyed. You might as well be eating cardboard. Here are some side effects of eating microwaved food:

. High blood pressure

. Anxiety

. Reproductive disorders

. Sleep disturbance

. Migraines

. Hair loss

. Heart disease

. Brain damage

. Dizziness

. Appendicitis

. Memory loss

. Stomach pains

. Cataracts

. Depression

. Cancer

. etc.

The magnetic field surrounding a microwave oven causes an abundance of health problems, as well, especially since some microwave radiation may leak from the microwave itself whilst it's still in use.

If you want to try an experiment, start watering your plants with water that's been heated inside a microwave for even a minute. Once you start watering your plants with the microwave-heated water, you'll find that your plants will start dying.

F.) Do not smoke. We all know that smoking in very detrimental to our health. Smoking will rob your brain of oxygen and is linked to cancer.

Smoking causes:

. Strokes

. Coronary heart disease

. Cardiovascular disease

. Damage of the blood vessels

. Lung disease

For women smoking can cause:

. Early delivery

. Stillbirth

. Low birth weight

. Sudden infant death syndrome

. ectopic pregnancy

. Orofacial clefts in infants

G.) Stop drinking alcohol and coffee, as they overload your liver and acidify your body. These drinks will dehydrate your body because they have a diuretic effect – meaning that they will cause the body to pass more liquid through urination. Here are some signs of dehydration:

. A dry mouth

. Weakness

. Headaches

. Dizziness

. Extreme fatigue

H.) Stop harbouring negative emotions such as anger, jealousy, hatred, envy and grudges, and replace them with loving thoughts instead. It's crucial for you to forgive people who've wronged you, as those negative emotions produce adrenaline and cortisol. Adrenaline is a hormone released from the adrenal gland and its major action is to prepare the body for "fight or flight". Adrenaline will make your heart beat irregularly.

Cortisol is a steroid hormone that regulates a wide range of vital processes throughout the body, including metabolism and immune response. It also has a very important role in helping the body respond to stress. But when produced for too long, it's going to impair your immune system. You can see for yourself that holding negative emotions or refusing to forgive people is counterproductive and will create diseases and disharmony in your body.

. Anger weakens your liver

. Sadness affects your lungs

. Anxiety affects your stomach

. Fear affects your kidneys

. Stress weakens your heart and brain

. But love brings peace and harmony

I.) You need to stop stressing yourself out. Stress produces adrenaline and cortisol, like I mentioned earlier. When stress is acute, your heart rate and blood pressure increase, but they return to normal once the acute stress has passed. If acute stress is repeatedly experienced or if your stress becomes chronic, it can cause damage to blood vessels and arteries. Stress wreaks havoc on your immune system.

Here are some physical symptoms of stress:

. Low energy

. Stomach upset

. Headaches

. Diarrhea

. Constipation

. Nausea

. Aches, pains, tense muscle

. Insomnia

. Frequent colds and infections

. Loss of sexual desire

. Chest pain and irregular heart beat

J.) Drink plenty of water. Your body uses water in all of its cells, organs and tissues to help regulate its temperature and maintain other bodily functions. Because your body loses water through breathing, sweating and digestion, it's vitally important for you to rehydrate by drinking water and eating foods which contain water, i.e., fruits. Other drinks will never replace water.

K.) Become more active. You can do simple exercises such as walking, light jogging, biking, etc... The key here, is not to do exercise until you're completely exhausted; just be active. Physical exercises facilitate the delivery of nutrients and facilitate the removal of toxins. Other benefits:

. Controls weight

. Combats health conditions and diseases

. Improves mood

. Boosts energy

. Promotes better sleep

. Puts the spark back into your sex life

. Can be fun and social

L.) You need to breathe fresh air. Fresh air helps the airwaves in your lungs to dilate more fully and improve the cleansing action of your lungs. When you exhale through your lungs, you release airborne toxins. Fresh air has been shown, as well, to help digest food more effectively, improve blood pressure and heart rate and strengthen the immune system, leading to an optimal health. You'll feel a lot happier and you will have more energy and a sharper mind.

Another good reason to get fresh air and walk in parks is because it's more toxic in our homes than outside. The toxicity created inside our houses is created due to

. cleaning products

. hairsprays

. deodorants

. perfumes

. electromagnetic frequencies

. wireless devices

. and electrical appliances.

This is what is called toxic-building syndrome, where the air quality in your home or office is so bad that it can actually affect the health of those inside. You might think that you're breathing clean air but, in fact, the air inside your home can have more than 900 harmful chemicals and organisms in it, which you simply cannot see. It's a good idea to spend time outdoors.

M.) Get sunlight exposure. Nothing is more important to us on Earth than the sun. Without the sun's heat and light, the Earth would be lifeless with nothing but ice-coated rocks. The sun gets our seas warm, steers our atmosphere, generates our weather patterns and provides energy to the growing green plants that produce the food and oxygen required for life on Earth. When natural sunlight hits the skin, it triggers the body's production of vitamin D. Vitamin D is also known as the sunshine vitamin. It's a crucial ingredient for overall health – it protects against inflammation, lowers high blood pressure, helps muscles, improves brain functionality and even protects against cancer. Vitamin D is very important and controls over 2,500 genes in our body.

Vitamin D:

. Enables you to absorb calcium and promotes bone growth.

. Makes muscles stronger and makes your lungs healthy

. The lower the vitamin D, the higher the blood pressure

. Regulates kidneys

. Protects you from cancer, diabetes, strokes and heart disease

You also receive vitamin D through your hair and eyes. Wearing sunglasses actually prevents your body from getting vitamin D through your eyes. Sun worshippers are also being warned that wearing sunglasses could increase the risk of skin cancer. Sunglasses make the brain think it's dark and this means you're not starting the natural process of tanning. You're more likely to burn and therefore at more of a risk of getting skin cancer. You also get photons from the sun. These photons will enter your body through your eyes and will be transformed into micro electricity that your brain will use for different functions. By wearing sunglasses, you prevent your eyes from absorbing photons. The sun provides a spectrum of light which is not replicable that enhances and maintains numerous processes in the brain. The sun doesn't give you cancer, as we've been brainwashed to believe. When you look at the past, our forefathers used to spend most of their time outdoors and there were no incidents of cancer. There is no need for you to fear the sun and, as a matter of fact, a lot of health issues are caused because of an extreme lack of sunlight.

It's now proven that a lack of sunlight can lead to osteoporosis, cancer and depression among other issues. And the SPF1 billion sunscreens we've been told to wear has now been proven to be a known carcinogen and actually causes skin cancer. Most people still have no idea about this, but the research is clear and it'll become common knowledge in the next few years.

Here are some carcinogens used in the sunscreen:

. benzophenone

. 4MBC

. avobenzone

. homosalate

. octocrylene

. and octinoxate to name a few.

Food companies which will use these ingredients will see their licenses revoked immediately but, somehow, you're allowed to use these on your skin. And as I told you before, when you put something on your skin, it goes directly into your bloodstream without filtering of any kind.

N.) You need enough sleep. Sleep plays a vital role in good health and wellbeing throughout your life. Getting enough quality sleep at the right times can help protect your mental health, physical health, quality of life and safety. During sleep, your body is working to support healthy brain functionality and maintain your physical health. As you drift off to sleep, your body begins its nightshift work: healing damaged cells, boosting your immune system, recovering from the day's activities and recharging your heart and cardiovascular system for the next day.

So now you can understand how sleep is vital but, above all, you need to sleep at night, as there's an important hormone called melatonin which is only releases at night when we sleep. People doing nightshifts on a permanent basis would be better off finding a daytime job. Melatonin is a very powerful antioxidant that fights

. inflammation

. promotes good sleep

. fights aging

. boosts the immune system

. and slows down the growth of certain types of cancer.

Melatonin is only released when you sleep in complete darkness. Do not sleep with the lights on.

O.) Eat a plant-based nutrition. For your body to work optimally, you need to give it the fuel it was designed for. The fuels for the human body are fruits, vegetables, legumes, grains, nuts and seeds. Plants are rich sources of many nutrients that are important for good health. They include unsaturated fats, vitamins, minerals, fibres and proteins. Yes, you read proteins correctly. We've been brainwashed to think that you can only get protein from animals. In fact, the human body doesn't even need animal protein but, rather, vegetal protein. Even the strongest and biggest land animal, the elephant, doesn't eat meat, but gets protein from the greens it eats everyday.

Here are some sources of protein that you can eat on a plant-based nutrition:

. Lentils

. Chickpeas

. Green peas

. Beans

. Seeds and nuts

. Hempseed

. Tofu

. Tempeh

. etc...

Sources of calcium for a plant-based nutrition:

. Broccoli

. Cabbage

. Okra

. Brussel sprouts

. Kale

. Spinach

. etc...

Sources of omega-3 fatty acids for a plant-based nutrition:

. Chia seeds

. Brussel sprouts

. Algae oil

. Hempseed

. Walnut

. Flaccid

. Perilla oil

Eating on a plant-based nutrition has been linked to a lower risk of obesity and many chronic diseases such as heart disease, type 2 diabetes, inflammation and cancer. People on a plant-based nutrition live much longer. They have longer life expectancies than meat eaters and grow older with fewer health issues. But why is that? Those on a plant-based nutrition tend to have:

- Healthier gut profiles, reduced abundance of pathogenic gut bacteria and greater abundance of protective species

- Lower blood pressure

- Lower incidents of heart disease

- Lower overall cancer incidents

- Lower risk of developing diabetes

That's a pretty impressive list of diseases that you can be protected against simply by adopting a plant-based nutrition. And it includes two of the top killers in western countries: heart disease and cancer.

Your average doctor will tell you that going plant-based will bring about a number of deficiencies, namely B12. The argument that people who don't consume animal products must have a B12 deficiency and endanger their health is not scientific and is misleading. There are billions of beneficial bacteria residing in our intestines and mouths, and they produce more than enough B12. The amount of vitamin B12 that a healthy person will require throughout their lifetime is actually very small. In addition, the liver can store B12 for many years and can recycle it, too. This is an explanation of as to why vegans eating a balanced diet almost never suffer from B12 deficiencies. But if your liver and intestines are congested, you may eventually develop a B12 deficiency, regardless of whether you're a meat eater, a vegetarian or a vegan. The common causes of a B12 deficiency are the antibiotics and other drugs which destroy the beneficial bacteria in our mouths and intestines.

P.) Eat less. It's a good idea to eat less, rather than more. 80% of our energy goes into digesting food. Your body can only cleanse and repair itself when it's not digesting food. In the same way, when you take your car to the mechanics, you can't drive it while it's being repaired. But in the world we're living in, we're really encouraged to eat multiple times a day. But as you can see, eating too frequently and too much will put a lot of burdens on your system.

Even when you're sick, at home or in the hospital, they'll subtly force you to eat by telling you that if you eat, you'll get more strength. But all of us have noticed that when we're not well, we lose our appetite. This isn't just a random fact. Your body is so intelligent that it doesn't want to spend 80% of its energy to digest food: it wants to use that energy to repair itself. That's what all the animals do when they're ill. They stop eating until they're well again. It's only human beings who don't listen to their bodies.

Fasting is the greatest healing tool, as it enables you to get rid of toxins. When you fast, you become less susceptible to disease. Fasting increases your degree of vitality and your intolerance to drugs. It helps repair and improve sleep and memory, and extend your lifetime, too. Fasting gives the body the opportunity to heal itself. There was once an experiment done with rats in which the researchers divided a number of them into two groups: one group was overfed, whereas the other group was fed less. By the end of the experiment, the researchers' results surprisingly revealed that the rats who were fed less lived up to 50% longer than the overfed rats. Now, what can you gather from that? The less you eat, the better you become – and there's plenty more science to back that up.

PART IV

CONCLUSION

In conclusion, I'll say that our bodies have been created perfectly. It's a self-healing machine, unlike the man-made devices. It doesn't need anything external like a replacement part, medication or anything along those lines. When we are ill, it's essentially self-inflicted. We create diseases for ourselves one day at a time by the way we eat, think and act. We are what we eat.

When you ask a doctor why we are sick, they'll give you three reasons. First, they'll tell you that it's just old age. This is untrue, as I was sick when I was younger but my health is optimal despite the fact that I'm much older. Secondly, they will tell you that it's genetic, but genetic problems only account for 5% of all problems. There's something called epigenetic, which means "above the genes." It essentially means that you can have bad genes but that it's the environment in which your cells live that triggers the gene's expression. This means that if you have defective genes and you eat the food designed for this body, these defective genes will stay dormant. That's why I've said that genetic issues only account for 5%. We need to stop blaming the genes for our bad health. It's the lifestyle that we adopt that will determine the gene expression. Thirdly, the doctors will tell you that they don't know the reason for us being sick. This is untrue, as I've told you that we become ill because of toxicity and deficiency.

We are responsible for our health – it's not the responsibility of our family members and certainly not the responsibility of our doctors. Throughout this book, I've been able to show you that we can live a disease-free life if we are able to make the necessary changes. We are not victims of circumstances but we are the masters who can create something good for ourselves.

I'll finish with a quote from Dr Alan Greenberg:

"As a retired physician, I can honestly say that, unless you are in a serious accident, your best chance of living to a ripe old age is to avoid doctors and hospitals and learn about nutrition, herbal medicine and other forms of natural medicine, unless you are fortunate enough to have a naturopathic physician available. Almost all drugs are toxic and are designed only to treat symptoms and not to cure anyone. Vaccines are highly dangerous, have never been adequately studied or proven to be effective, and have a poor risk/reward ratio. Most surgery is unnecessary and most textbooks of medicine are inaccurate and deceptive.

Almost every disease is said to be idiopathic (without known cause) or genetic – although this is untrue. In short, our mainstream medical system is hopelessly inept and/or corrupt. The treatment of cancer and degenerative diseases is a national scandal. The sooner you learn this, the better off you will be.

FINIS

Please visit my website:www.oliviermankondo.com and learn more about my "weight loss and wellness program"

ME & MY WIFE: THE CHANGE

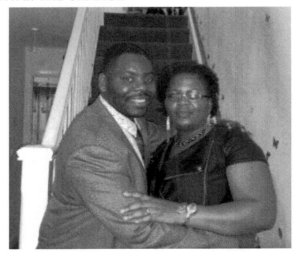

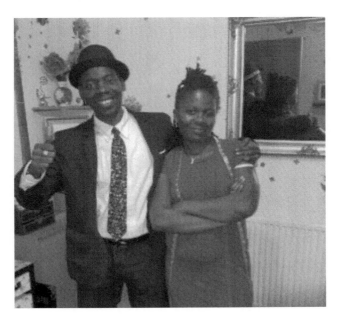

MY BROTHER: THE CHANGE

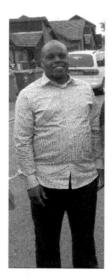

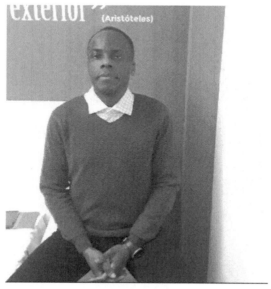

Printed in Poland
by Amazon Fulfillment
Poland Sp. z o.o., Wrocław